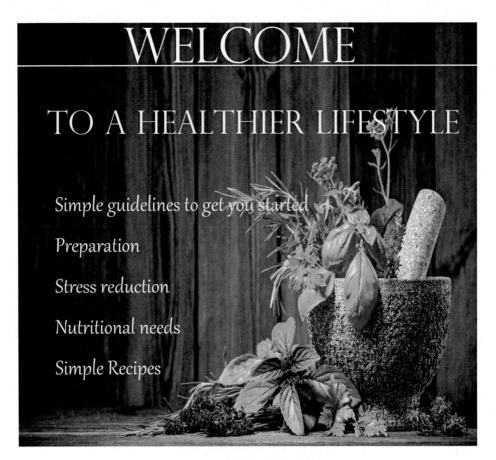

WELCOME

TO A HEALTHIER LIFESTYLE

Simple guidelines to get you started

Preparation

Stress reduction

Nutritional needs

Simple Recipes

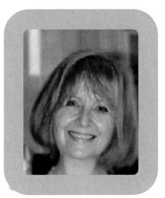

D1304321

Gloria Coppola, Lifestyle Specialist

Certified Health & Lifestyle Coach

<u>Acknowledgments</u>

I would like to thank my parents who showed me how to put love in cooking. We spent countless hours in the kitchen each Saturday preparing weekend meals. Every Saturday morning Dad and I would go to the fresh markets in Little Italy, NY.

The holidays were fun too! For weeks we would cook. When we got to cooking some pies, Dad would say "More cinnamon and nutmeg Gloria"? I'd smile and say YES! Mom would laugh and shake her head. The kitchen always smelled of some great spices and herbs and olive oil!

Next, I want to thank my health- coaching clients who continue to give me the motivation to find delicious, easy and healthy options you can enjoy in life that won't stress your budget or consume your time.

To David Wolfe, raw foodist. I love your nutrition classes. You continue to amaze me with your knowledge and passion.

Mark Reinfeld, author of Vegan Fusion. I never new raw vegan could taste so good!

David Sandoval, author of the Green Foods Bible you rebooted my health and inspired me to eat more Green Super Foods! My health has greatly improved.

In addition I must give credit and thanks to 3 lovely ladies who were my chefs at the retreats I host yearly. Meg, Elska and Alex you truly inspired me!

Lastly, The Tuscany Cooking School who inspired me to have fun cooking again!! Thank you everyone!

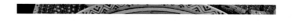

Dedication

Betsy Griffith, I never met you personally, RIP. It was your daughter who shared this recipe with me while I was writing this book. I just new it was a message from you. I also knew it was a message for all of us as we go through life. Thank you for writing it in your cookbook and now I shall pass it along!

If you can't cook
Anonymous

2 lbs. of hugs
1 lb. of kisses
2 warm glances
4 tsp. of cheery smiles

When days are dark and smiles rare, mix a little of this and that with generous sprinklings of beaming smiles and happiness will be found always in your kitchen.

Introduction

Welcome! Growing up Italian I spent many days in the kitchen with my parents. Each Saturday we would go to the fresh markets to get our produce, cheese, grains and fresh Italian bread and pastries. I loved the smell of olive oil and garlic sautéing in the kitchen. It is still one of my favorites!

This year I went to cooking school in Tuscany, Italy and a side trip to Greece where my passion for cooking was sparked once again.

I created this guide to inspire you! I want to help you find a love for cooking while taking simple steps to get healthier! Enjoy the journey!

Today, our processed foods are creating many unnecessary health symptoms and obesity. My contribution will provide you some information to help you make some simple changes that I hope you will enjoy and pass on to others.

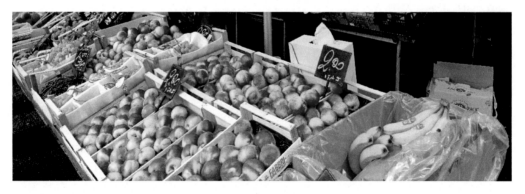

PS. I will be posting a few pictures from Italy and Greece too!

Table of contents

Throughout the booklet you will find Journal Pages to chart your progress and keep a diary to celebrate your success.

Try these suggestions for 10 days, 30 days or more!

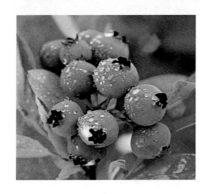

Section 1

Let's get started

It's a lifestyle — not a marathon — no need to rush
by changing everything all at once.

Let's start with you!

Create a space in your schedule where you will have time to
do something for yourself.

As your guide and coach I want you to be successful. I've been
helping people for 30 yrs. and I know it takes time to
accomplish realistic goals. Therefore, I want you to start this
journey in a manner that suits you. You will be more able to
continue to make healthier choices each day but you must be
ready!

Your lifestyle can be anything you desire!

Ask yourself what is most important to you?

Health? Weight loss?

Easy recipes for the family

A stress free life

Energy for exercise

Follow my suggestions for 30 days consistently!

Once you get on the right path, you will choose how you want to continue.

Perhaps you will become vegetarian? Maybe you will give up caffeine forever?

You might love cooking so much you will write your own cookbook!

I might even see you on the news for winning a marathon ☺

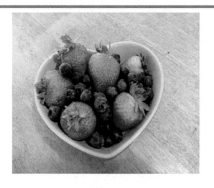

Start Here!

Over the course of approximately 5-10 days

Begin to remove the following from your daily diet.

- Processed foods

- Soda and all caffeine

- Sugar

- Avoid Fast Foods

- Dairy

- Increase your water intake.

- Then let's get you started with healthier meal options.

- Try going vegetarian or vegan for at least 10 days.

- Use the Journal pages to track your progress.

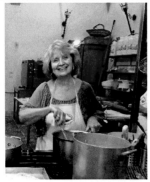

What do you need?

Tuscany Cooking School

- A positive mindset

- Organic Fresh Fruit & Organic Veggies

- Lots of water

- Support of family or friends

- Plastic containers and zip lock bags for easy storage of meals

- Food Processor, vita mixer or nutri bullet

- Basic condiments, fresh herbs

- Organic Olive oil and/or organic coconut oil

- A progress journal, which I've included here for your convenience.

- Take your before and after pictures too!

BASIC CONDIMENTS

I prefer fresh organic herbs whenever possible.
If you are purchasing dried herbs do your best to find organic herbs. The list will help you with the ingredients you will need for many of the recipes in this guide.

1. Basil
2. Parsley
3. Himalayan Sea salt
4. Rosemary
5. Cayenne
6. Cumin
7. Oregano
8. Curry
9. Pepper
10. Garlic
11. Onion
12. Celery
13. Turmeric
14. Cinnamon
15. Thyme
16. Fennel
17. Ginger

NOTES: _____

_____

_____

Goals - write them down

Weight: _____   _____

Health Goals: _____

_____

_____

Exercise: _____

_____

Target Date: _____

Notes: _____

_____

_____

_____

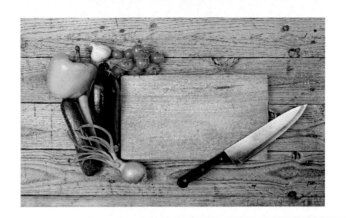

Set yourself up for success

Be prepared and organized

I love having great kitchen tools
1. Sharp Knife
2. Cutting boards
3. Lemon Squeezer
4. Sharp peeler
5. Food Processor
6. Spiralizer, Mandolin Slicer
7. 2 Cutting boards
8. Small bowls
9. Blender or Nutri Bullet

Use organic foods and herbs only
Grass fed meats & hormone free

PH-balanced water 7.0 or higher for alkalinity. Filtration systems are available that will alkaline your water.

Set aside time to prepare healthier foods. I like to prepare a few on the weekends. Midweek I choose recipes that take 30 minutes or less.

Notes: _____

<u>SHOPPING LIST</u>

1. Fresh organic fruit
   a. _____
   b. _____
   c. _____
   d. _____
2. Organic Veggies
   a. _____
   b. _____
   c. _____
   d. _____
3. Organic Spices
   a. _____
   b. _____
   c. _____
   d. _____

4. Apothe Cherry
5. Fresh Ginger
6. Activated Barley
7. Raw Organic Wraps

8. _____

9. _____

Flours: Almond flour, coconut flour
Nuts: Cashew, Almonds, pumpkin seeds, sunflower seeds, pecans
Meats: Grass fed, hormone free, antibiotic free
Oils: Organic coconut oil, olive oil

Recommended Organic Vegetables and Fruits

1. Broccoli
2. Cauliflower
3. Cabbage
4. Zucchini
5. Avocado
6. Berries
7. Squash
8. Red Pepper
9. Apples
10. Spinach
11. Sprouts
12. Beets
13. Celery
14. Cucumber
15. Fennel
16. Kale
17. Collards
18. Mushrooms
19. Arugula
20. Watermelon
21. Asparagus
22. Brussel sprouts
23. Turnips

NOTES: _____

_____

_____

Got Cravings?

Stress, emotions and an unhealthy gut all lead to cravings

Sugar Cravings? This may be caused by a fluctuation in blood sugar levels. There are also other factors as well, including parasites that feed on sugar. You may also have a deficiency in minerals like chromium, sulphur, phosphorus and tryptophan

- Substitute candy for fruit that is low in sugar like berries.
- Eat more vegetables with fiber like Broccoli, cauliflower
- Legumes
- Cinnamon

Chocolate cravings? These cravings are usually related to a deficiency in magnesium.
- Nuts, seeds, leafy greens
- Raw cacao

Salt cravings? Your adrenal glands may be stressed and the salt helps you cope with stress. It may also be a deficiency in Chloride and silicon

- Celery
- Seaweed
- Cashews, seeds
- Stress management and meditation

Cheese craving? Your body needs some healthy fatty acids. Omega 3's
- Raw walnuts
- Wild Salmon
- Flax seeds, hemp or chia seeds

Cravings can also be related to dehydration! Drink more water! Statistics suggest 80% of people are dehydrated*

* www.active.com/nutrition

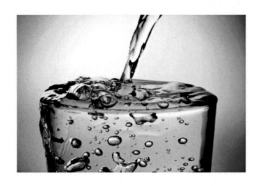

HYDRATION

Drinking enough water daily is important for everyone. Most people are dehydrated and don't even know it. Room temperature is recommended vs. ice cold.

"Hydration is important because the body is comprised mostly of water, and the proper balance between water and electrolytes in our bodies really determines how most of our systems function, including nerves and muscles," says Larry Kenney, PhD, a professor of physiology and kinesiology at Penn State. ~ Web MD

Once you are thirsty you are already dehydrated. Drink at least ½ your body weight in ounces daily. This is especially important if you are exercising or detoxing your body.

I like to recommend 5 cups of plain hot water daily!
This is an old ayurvedic remedy to help cleanse the lymphatic system. It helps eliminate cravings and aids in weight loss.

1 cup upon awakening, 1 before each meal and 1 30 minutes prior to bedtime.

Notes:

_____

_____

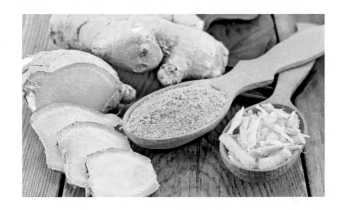

Caffeine withdrawal remedy
Ginger Cinnamon Tea

1. Fresh Ginger
2. Cinnamon Sticks
3. Green apple

This simple remedy will help you eliminate caffeine without headaches and cravings and provide energy, boost your metabolism and reduce sugar cravings.

Directions:

Brew a Ginger, Cinnamon Tea.
1-quart water
Place several slices of ginger in your pot of water.
Add a cinnamon stick or 2.
Boil.

Serve a hot cup of ginger cinnamon tea.
Eat 1 apple.

You will be amazed how easily it is to eliminate caffeine withdrawals. Try it!

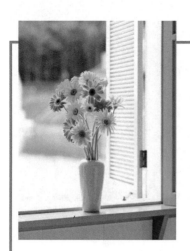

JOURNAL NOTES
Keep track of your progress
What foods are you learning to like
How are you feeling as the weeks go by
following this simple plan?

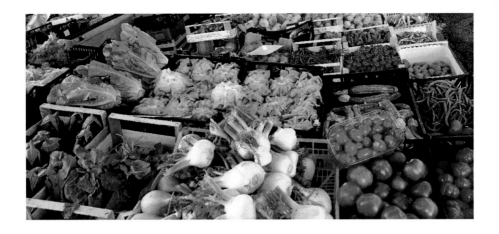

Buy organic, fresh, local vegetables when you have the opportunity! You'll find the flavors pop and the quality will make all the difference in the meals you prepare!

When vegetables have a chance to ripen before harvesting, the nutritional value is much higher! Buy Local! Start an herbal garden!

Try new things! As you start this journey, you may find your tastes buds change too! Explore! You just might be surprised how many delicious options out there are waiting for you….go ahead, give something new a chance.

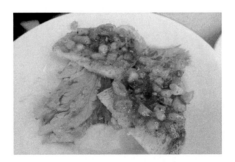

Try some fresh bruschetta! Easy to make. Dice plum tomatoes; add fresh basil, minced garlic! Sprinkle some sea salt and black pepper. Serve on toasted bread! YUM

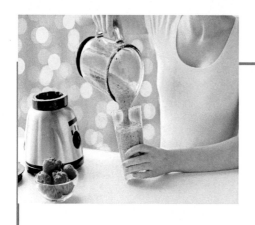

Section 2

Smoothies & Juicing

Great for anytime of the day

Easy and convenient

Packed full of nutrients & flavorful

Have fun mixing veggies and fruits!

Optional additions:

Raw Cacao- antioxidant

Maca - Rich in B Vitamins, Women's health

Chia – Omega 3

Spirulina – 65 % protein, Amino acids & Omega's

Kamut – Anti aging, Amino Acids, Lipids, Zinc

Rice Bran Soluble – Protein, Minerals & Vitamins

Goji berries – Beta Carotene, Healthy skin

Hemp seeds – Omega's

Notes:

_____

_____

_____

Coconut Green Smoothie

1. 1 Banana
2. 1 apple sliced
3. 1 teaspoon coconut oil
4. 1 cup of kale, remove stems
5. ½ cup coconut milk
6. ½ ripe avocado
7. Blend well with ice

Mango Coconut Smoothie

1. 1 ripe banana
2. 2 ripe honey mangos, pitted and peeled
3. ½ cup coconut milk
4. 1 juice of a lime
5. Blend with ice

BlackBerry Spinach Smoothie

1. 2 cups of fresh blackberries
2. 2 cups of spinach, remove stems
3. 1 teaspoon raw local honey
4. 1 stalk of celery
5. ½ cucumber, peeled
6. ¼ cup Goji berries
7. Blend with ice until smooth

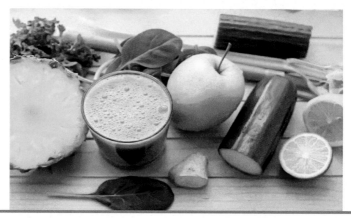

There are lots of fancy juicers available however I prefer to juice my ingredients, in my Nutri Bullet or Vita Mixer. I know I will be getting all the value of every nutrient and the pulp gives me the necessary fiber required daily too.

It's easy. It's simple. It's delicious and nutritious!

Start simple

1. 1 cup of pineapple or 1 banana
2. 1 cup of kale, stems remove
3. 1 apple, diced
4. ½ cup of coconut milk or almond milk or coconut water
5. ½ cup of ice
6. 1 stalk of celery diced
7. ½ cucumber
8. 1 cup spinach

Directions: Put all the ingredients in your blender until smooth. Serve Immediately.

Try adding different veggies and fruits daily. Experiment with flavors by adding cinnamon, lemon juice, fresh ginger.

Notes: _____
_____

Detox Green Juice

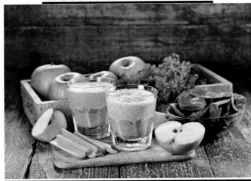

1. 2 stalks of organic celery
2. 1 apple sliced
3. 1 cup of kale, stems removed
4. ½ cup of spinach
5. 1 cup of parsley
6. 1 fresh organic lemon
7. 1 finger of fresh ginger sliced
8. 1 cup of cold water

Optional: 1 teaspoon Maca for energy, stress reduction & hormonal balance

Directions: Put all your ingredients in your Nutri Bullet or Vitamixer and blend until smooth. Serve immediately

Notes:

_____

_____

Always choose organic vegetables and fruits especially when you are detoxing.

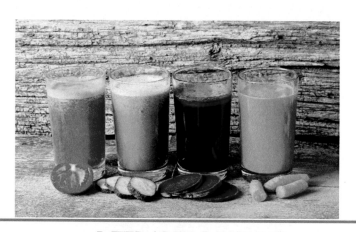

MIX AND MATCH
Have fun creating!
Beet & Kale Juice

1 medium orange, peeled and diced

3 kale leaves, remove stems

1 medium apple, cut into wedges

1 medium carrot, peeled

1 large beet, peeled and diced

1 1-inch piece peeled fresh ginger

Ice cubes (optional)

Blend well in your Vita Mixer or Nutri Bullet.

If you prefer to use a Juicer (like a champion juicer etc., it is up to you)

Optional: 1 Orange vs. carrot

Beets are great for your blood. Eat from the rainbow because every color fruit or vegetable directly keeps various parts of our body healthier!

Nutrition Bonus: Vitamin A (80% daily value), Vitamin C (38% dv) – EatingWell.com

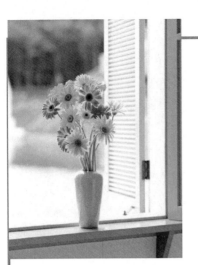

JOURNAL PAGE

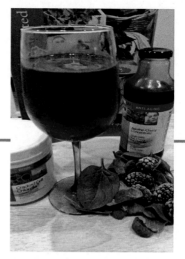

Blackberry avocado smoothie

Energy and hormonal balance

- 1.5 cups of coconut water, coconut milk or almond milk
- 1 cup frozen blackberries rich in bioflavonoids.
- 1/2 cup raw spinach. Rich in antioxidants and high source of vitamin A and B and C.
- 1/2 avocado. Healthy monosaturated fat.
- 1 tsp. Maca. Rich in B vitamins. Women's health and moods. Good for libido. 1 tsp. cinnamon helps lower blood sugar
- 1/2 tsp. vanilla. Antioxidant. Aphrodisiac.
- 1 tbsp. Chia. High in omega 3 fat acids.
- 1 tbsp. raw cacao. Magnesium and other essential minerals.
- 1 tbsp. cracked cell chlorella. Great source of protein. Richest source of chlorophyll. Natural detoxification
- 1 tbsp. Apothe cherry. Melatonin. Healthy joint function. Anti aging.
- Notes:_____

_____

Resources: www.longevitywarehouse.com

Acai & Berry Bowl

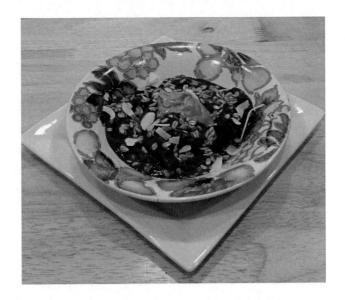

- Absolutely one of my favorites! You can blend it with many different options.
- 1-2 packets frozen acai. **Acai** contain antioxidants, fiber and heart-healthy fats.
- Add blueberry, raspberry, strawberry or blackberry if desired. 1/2 cup
- ½ frozen banana
- Add ½ cup coconut water, almond milk, or coconut milk.
- Mix in a Vita mixer or nutri bullet until smooth and blended well
- Top with Granola, shredded coconut, banana, peanut or almond butter, raw cacao chips
- Optional: You can also blend spinach, Spirulina, maca, cinnamon etc.
    - Spirulina is natures vitamin and contains protein

Notes:

_____

_____

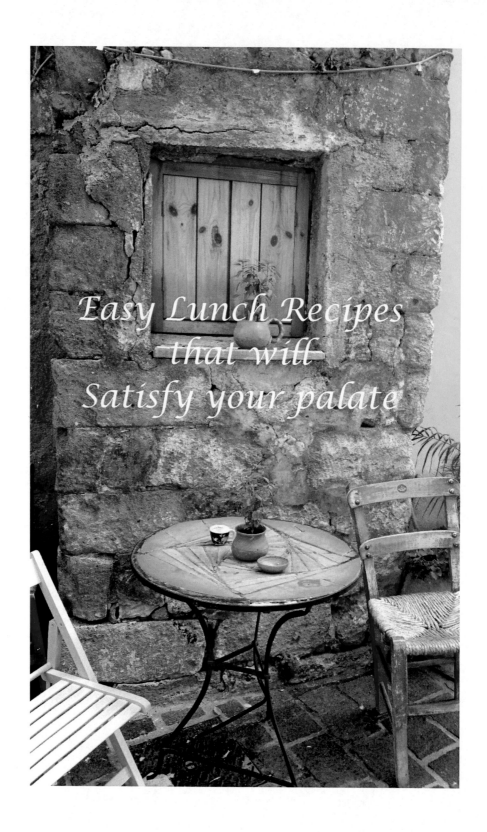

Easy Lunch Recipes
that will
Satisfy your palate

Eating Healthier

You are making wiser choices now!
Let's talk Avocados! A healthy fat!

Avocado can help you meet the dietary guidelines of the American Heart Association, which are to eat a diet that is low to moderate in fat. The fats should be primarily unsaturated and low in saturated fats and cholesterol. The AHA recommends limiting saturated fats to less than 7 percent of your total daily intake of fats.

A 1 oz. serving of avocado contains 0.5 grams saturated fat and is cholesterol free, making it a good choice to help you meet the dietary guidelines.

Avocado helps support your immune system, cardiovascular, teeth and bones as well as digestive system and muscle development.

Contains: Magnesium, Zinc, C, Copper and Riboflavin.

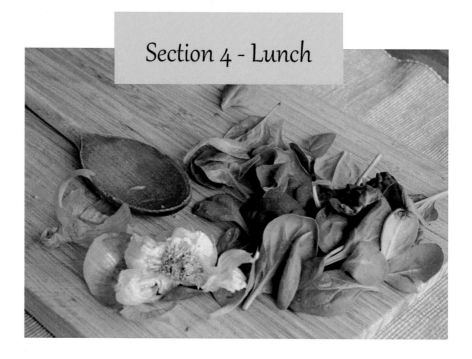

Section 4 - Lunch

Spinach is the storehouse for many phytonutrients that promote health and have disease prevention properties.

Fresh spinach leaves are a rich source of several vital anti-oxidant vitamins including A and C, lutein and beta-carotene. Together these compounds help act as protective scavengers against oxygen derived free radicals and reactive oxygen species that play a healing role in aging and various disease processes. Spinach leaves are an excellent source of Vitamin K, as well.

100 grams of spinach contains about 25% of daily iron intake and is one of the richest green leafy vegetables.

Recipe:
Sautee spinach in some organic olive oil and minced garlic. Easy to prepare and delicious. Add fresh lemon juice or Himalayan salt if desired.

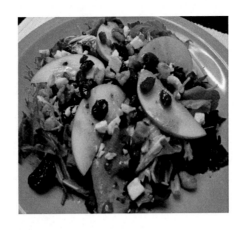

SPINACH & APPLE SALAD

High in Vitamin K, A, C and niacin.

3 cups of organic spinach
- Rinse and dry
- Remove stems
- 1 green apple sliced

Optional toppings: Greek olives, feta cheese, apples, cranberries, pecans, walnuts, Sundried tomatoes, etc.

Drizzle with a balsamic vinegar

Notes:

_____
_____
_____
_____
_____

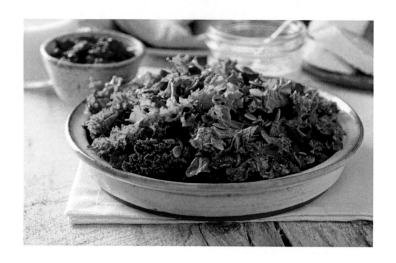

<u>KALE SALAD</u>

- Rinse your organic kale. Remove excess water. Remove the stems.
- Fold the leaf in half and chop in small to medium pieces.
- Prepare ¼ cup organic olive oil and 1 squeezed fresh lemon. Add Sea salt to taste. ¼ tsp. to ½ tsp. of raw honey. Mix it up.
- Drizzle on your kale a little at a time while massaging your kale. Yes it breaks down the bitterness. It will turn a bright green.
- Add diced red pepper, avocado, artichoke hearts, sundried tomato, cranberries or pecans etc.,
- Get creative!
- Optional: Sprinkle with sesame seeds

Nearly 3 grams of protein. 2.5 grams of fiber (which helps manage blood sugar and makes you feel full) Vitamins A, C, and K (Web MD)

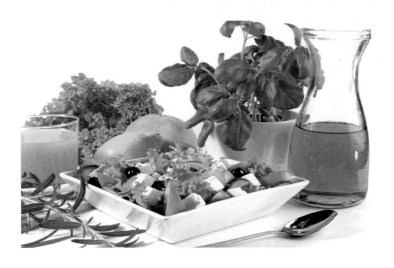

<u>Greek Salad with home made dressing</u>

1 bag organic Mixed Greens
1 red onion, sliced
1 cucumber, diced
½ cup black kalamata olives, pitted
1 tomato diced
½ cup artichoke hearts

<u>Dressing</u>
½ cup olive oil, the juice of 1 lemon and 1 teaspoon red wine vinegar
½ clove garlic, minced
½ teaspoon oregano
Shake it up

Top with ½ cup crumbled feta cheese

Toss the vegetables and salad greens in a large bowl.
Combing the dressing and blend well. Toss and sprinkle with cheese (optional)

Zucchini Salad

1 organic zucchini carefully slice lengthwise with a mandolin slicer. ¼ inch
2 cups organic mixed greens 50/50 mix with spinach
1 organic tomato diced or grape tomatoes
½ cucumber diced

Fresh Basil
Dash of sea salt and pepper

Dressing
Drizzle balsamic vinegar

Optional
Feta cheese
Red pepper
Artichoke hearts
Olives
Grapes
Pecans, chopped

Notes:

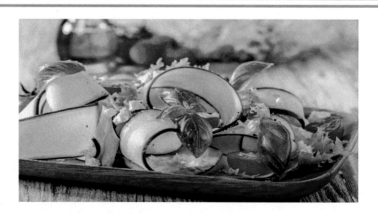

Grilled Avocado

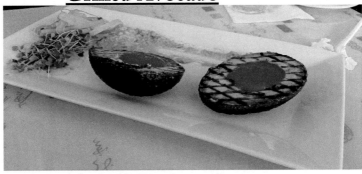

1 organic avocado cut in half. Remove pit
Slice lines across (as in photo).
Place on grill or frying pan to warm

Red pepper sauce

1 red pepper or roasted pepper
(Optional choice of tomato vs. pepper)
1 clove garlic
½ tsp. olive oil
½ teaspoons Italian seasoning
Dash of sea salt

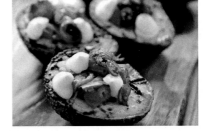

Optional: ½ red chili pepper,
Blend in food processor. Warm

Add red pepper sauce inside avocado
Optional: Mozzarella, rosemary, olives

Serve with a side of sprouts, hummus or salad

Notes: _____

_____

HUMMUS

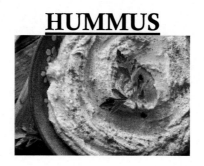

Middle Eastern recipe that is easy to make anytime.

I've substituted cauliflower for chickpeas and it's delicious. Experiment even with zucchini!

- 2 cups Chickpeas, soak overnight or at least 2 hrs. Drain and rinse. Optional: Roast them a bit for a nuttier taste before blending.
- ½ organic Lemon juice
- 3 tbsps. Organic Olive Oil
- 1 clove Garlic
- Dash of Sea Salt to taste.
- ½ tsp. black pepper
- Optional – roasted red pepper, spinach

Substitution: ½ head steamed cauliflower vs. chickpeas

I like to add different vegetables in my hummus. So get creative and blend them up!

Throw your ingredients in your Vita Mixer/food processor and blend until smooth. Adjust the consistency by adding drops of olive oil or lemon juice.

Notes: _____

_____

RAW WRAPS

- Purchase in health food store or online -Raw Zucchini/Apple Wraps (Vegan, Gluten Free, Organic). You can also substitute lettuce
- ½ sliced and peeled cucumber
- ½ cup spinach
- ½ ripened avocado
- 1 roasted red pepper
- Place ingredients in the wrap.
- Optional: Dash of Himalayan Sea salt, Dijon mustard
- Roll up and enjoy

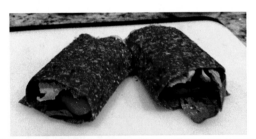

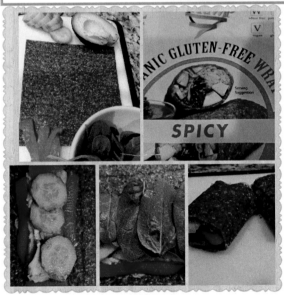

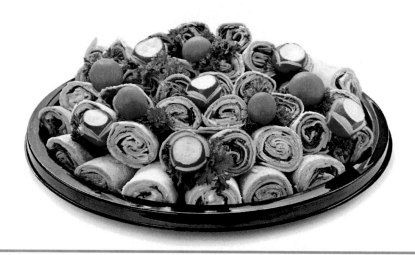

<u>Wraps are quick, easy and delicious</u>
Substitute lettuce leaves for your wrap if you prefer

Favorite Ingredients:

- Hummus
- Sprouts
- Spinach, lettuce
- Roasted red pepper
- Avocado
- Dijon mustard, olive oil, balsamic vinegar
- Grilled veggies, eggplant, onion, bell pepper, etc.
- Cheese optional
- Roll them up and enjoy!

Optional: Ezekiel Wraps (health food store or your frozen food section at your grocers)

Notes: _____

_____

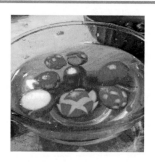

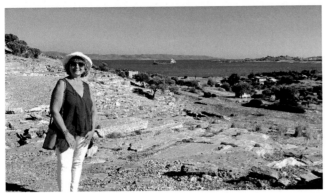

Greetings from Greece

I hope you are enjoying your simple lifestyle changes and noticing that you are feeling better, gaining more energy and loving your new choices.

Remember to journal how you are feeling, what are the next steps you would like to take and what are your next goals? It's all a journey, so enjoy it!

Prepare for some great dessert and snacks made from fruits and veggies! That's right! They taste amazing and I hope you enjoy what's coming up! Of course, after dinner. However, if you are like me you might like to do dessert first sometimes ☺

Let's get moving first ....

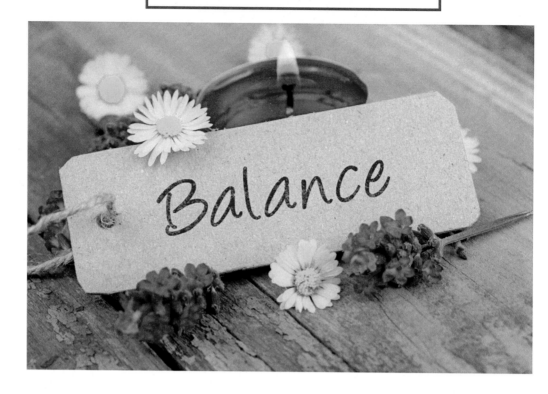

Everything is about balance! The only way we can stick to any lifestyle program is if we create balance in our life.

80% nutrition
20% exercise

Yoga, walking, aerobics, weight lifting, whatever is your choice, consistently do it at least 3 times a week.

Rest is equally important.
Get to bed by 10pm for a deep restful sleep

Massage is great to reduce stress
A monthly massage minimally will keep your body fine tuned.

Exercise

Let's get moving! Gently, slowly and make it fun. Your body will love it too! Moving your body helps your lymphatic system work more efficiently too. This is the system in your body where toxins move through.

YOGA

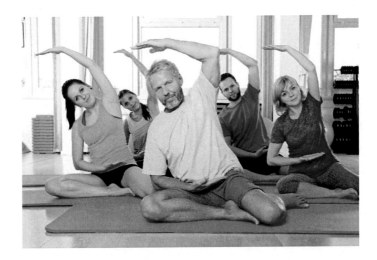

There are many styles of yoga, however I suggest starting with a simple basic class like Hatha yoga. Start stretching easily, learn how to breathe and relax. Calm your mind, gain more mindfulness and feel fabulous!

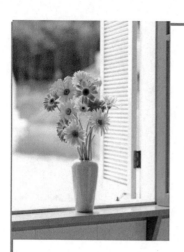

<u>JOURNAL PAGE</u>

Massage

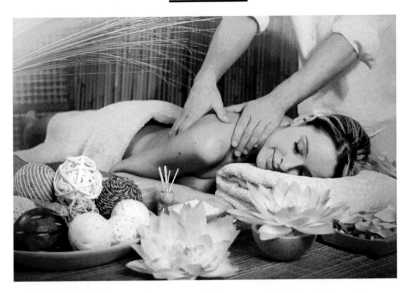

Did you know massage could help your body function better?
Gentle massage helps the lymphatic system. The lymphatic system is
the place where all the byproducts in our body move through.

Relaxing your nervous system helps you think clearer, provides feel
good hormones and relaxes your muscles too.

Massage does not have to be deep to be beneficial.
Allow yourself to be nurtured. You are making some great changes in
your life for your body and now your mind too.

Massage is also great when trying to lose weight, reducing stress,
balancing emotions and improving circulation.

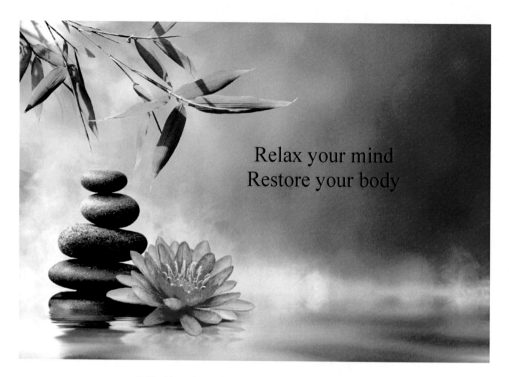

Relax your mind
Restore your body

Meditation for stress reduction

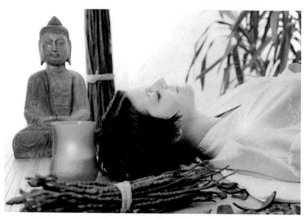

Find a comfortable place. Sit or lay down. Optional soft music may be played.
Breathe deeply 30 breaths into your belly and exhale through your mouth.
Relax your muscles
Let your thoughts float off and relax your mind
Begin relaxing for 5 minutes and increase to 30 minutes
Just let go

FRESH AIR

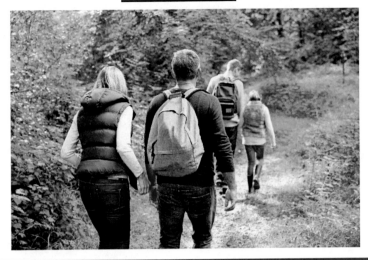

Get out in nature and go for walks 3-5 times a week
Start with 15 minutes and build it up for as long as you like.

Restful Sleep

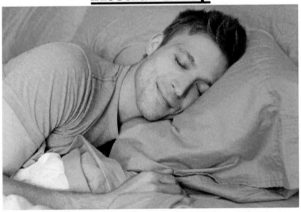

Go to bed by 10pm for a deep restorative sleep
It's important to get into deep cycles of sleep so your body can
naturally detox nightly and regenerate
Wake up more refreshed

I recommend 1 tablespoon of Apothe Cherry (Tart cherry drink)
mixed with hot or cold water 30 minutes prior to bedtime.

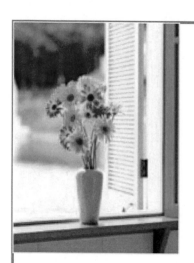

JOURNAL PAGE

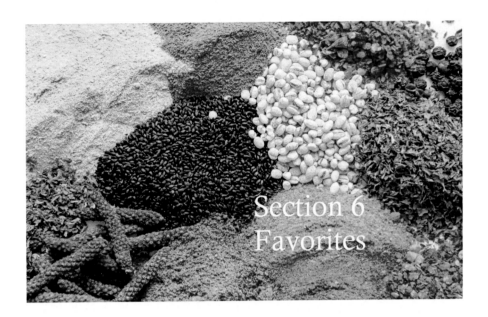

Section 6
Favorites

Let's create some more healthy options!

I love Quinoa! Cooking with quinoa is a lot easier than you might think! It's very versatile too, hot or cold. This amazing gluten free, vegan ancient protein, packs in the nutrition with flavors.

"Quinoa is native to Bolivia and is relative to Swiss chard, spinach and beets. What's more, it comes in three varieties (whole grain white, red and black). Just 1 cup contains 8g of protein, 5g of fiber, 30% magnesium, 19% DV folate and heart healthy Omega 3 fatty acids" ~ Ancient Grains

Quinoa is actually a seed, not a grain by the way and provides 9 essential amino acids necessary for good health.

I started using quinoa when I realized the starch in rice was not the best choice for my body. I especially love the nutty flavor of the tricolor quinoa. It's a great substitute without all the starch.

Winter Harvest Quinoa

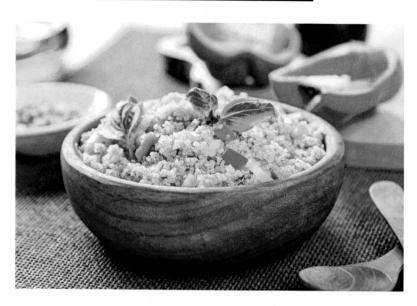

Great for breakfast or anytime!

Ingredients

- 1 cup of quinoa. Soak prior and rinse well
- 2 cups of apple cider
- 1 tsp. freshly grated ginger
- ¼ tsp. Himalayan salt
- ¼ cup coconut milk, unsweetened (not canned)
- 1 cup butternut squash, peeled, seeded and diced
- Optional: Fresh blueberries with a dash of cinnamon are great for breakfast
- 1/3 cup of water
- 2 tbsp. pecans, chopped (optional)
- 2 tbsp. dried cranberries

Instructions

- Place quinoa in medium size pot. Add apple cider, ginger and salt. Cook on medium heat until it boils. Simmer
- 1/3 cup water and butternut squash. Cook until tender
- Place squash in food processor, blend until smooth
- Flush quinoa. Whip in squash and coconut milk. Cook uncovered on low heat for 5 mins.
- Serve. Top with cranberries, pecans or cinnamon

Quinoa Soup

___Ingredients___

- 1 cup quinoa. Soak, rinse and drain before cooking.
- 1 cup cooked wild rice or brown rice
- 1 cup soak, rinsed, drained chickpeas
- 1 cup kale, remove the stems and dice
- 1 small onion, diced
- 1 clove garlic, minced
- ¼ cup parsley, chopped
- ½ teaspoon Himalayan salt
- ½ teaspoon black pepper
- Optional: ½ red chili pepper, diced for some extra kick

1. Cook rice and quinoa according to package
2. Cook vegetables in 3 cups water. Add onion, garlic, salt, parsley and pepper
3. Drain rice and quinoa and put into a large bowl
4. Add veggies and enough broth to cover the ingredients
5. Stir well
6. Top with fresh parsley or basil

NOTES: _____

_____

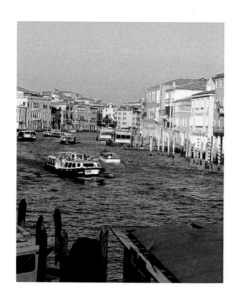

Italy inspired me! The foods were delicious! It reminded me of all the great foods I had as a kid, growing up near little Italy, NYC.

The ingredients were so pure and fresh; nothing I ate bothered my stomach. Pick and choose your ingredients wisely for best flavors.

FRESH IS BEST!

If you ever have the chance to go to cooking school in Tuscany, do it! It was so much fun!

I've also been studying with other chefs and learning how to turn cashews into cheese, for those that are dairy free and it is surprisingly delicious. If you are gluten free or just want to try something different I now make my pasta with zucchini. Check out my faux raw marinara sauce coming up next with zucchini pasta.

Buon Appetito!

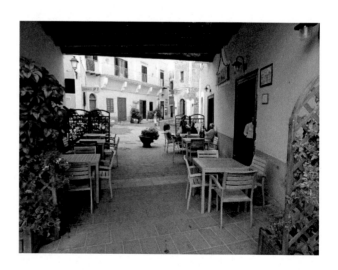

Roasted Red Pepper Sauce

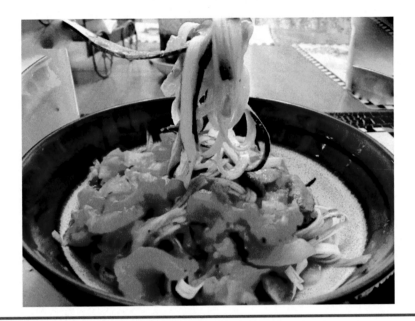

- 2 large roasted red peppers
- 1 clove of garlic
- ½ teaspoon olive oil
- ½ teaspoon Italian herbal seasoning
- ¼ teaspoon Himalayan salt
- Pepper (optional)

1. Place all ingredients in a food processor
2. Blend quickly. Leave it a little bit chunky
3. Heat if desired. I use it at room temperature with my raw zucchini (see recipes next page).

This is a great replacement when making a tomato based marinara sauce.

NOTES:_____

_____

Zucchini Pasta

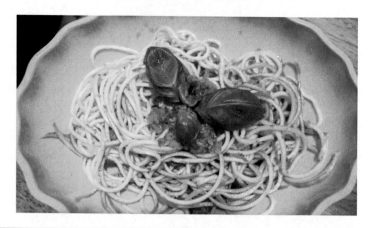

You will need a Spiralizer to make the raw zucchini spaghetti

- 1-2 organic zucchini. Peel and Spiralize
- If you prefer, you may warm it up lightly by quickly steaming or blanching. If you add some coconut oil while steaming the zucchini, it will add another dimension to the taste.
- Top with the roasted red pepper sauce
- Add Fresh Basil
- Optional: Dash of Himalayan salt or cheese
- Optional: The raw zucchini pasta is also delicious with a guacamole or pesto sauce

NOTES: _____

_____

Zucchini Fries

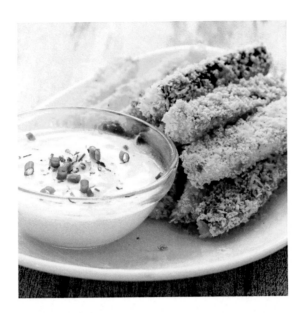

- 2-3 large organic zucchini
- Slice zucchini into wedges
- Coat with activated barley or bread crumbs
- Fry in coconut oil until golden

Dips: Greek yogurt with lime juice and cayenne
Marinara sauce

NOTES: _____

_____

Zucchini Pizza Bites

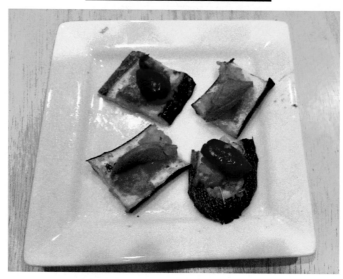

- 2-3 large organic zucchini
- Wash the skin and leave it on
- Carefully Slice lengthwise on a mandolin about ¼ to ½ inch thick
- Drizzle organic olive oil on the slices
- Add Italian herbal seasoning
- Add diced tomato or roasted red pepper
- Place on a pizza pan. Bake at 350 degrees until tender, approximately 20-30 minutes
- Top with fresh basil, olives or nutritional yeast
- Optional: Cheese
- Cut into bite sizes

NOTES: _____

_____

Vegetarian Beet Reuben

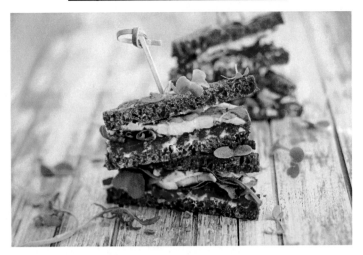

- Sprouted Grain Bread, Pumpernickel or Sourdough lightly toasted
- 1 ripe organic avocado
- 3 small beets cooked and sliced
- Swiss cheese, manchego cheese melted or any cheese of your choice
- 1 teaspoon spicy mustard, spread on bread. Mayonnaise optional
- Sprouts
- Optional: Sauerkraut

Layer ingredients on your choice of bread

NOTES: _____

_____

Cucumber Sushi

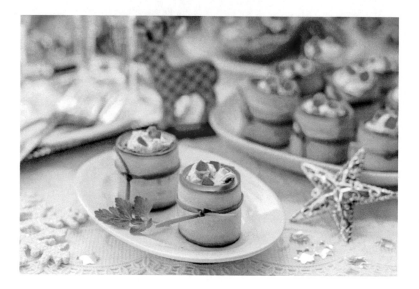

- 1 Organic English Cucumber. Slice lengthwise about ¼ inch thick

FILLING

- Goat cheese
- 2 teaspoons fresh dill
- 1/8 teaspoon Himalayan salt
- Red pepper strips
- Avocado
- Tomato
- Olives
- Optional: Cayenne pepper

Mix goat cheese dill and salt
Spread cheese mixture on the cucumber slices
Add your choice of other ingredients
Roll them up
Sprinkle with cayenne pepper
Use a tooth pic, cucumber skins sliced thinly or green ribbon to securely close

NOTES: _____

_____

Broccoli Soup

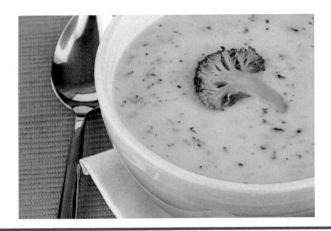

- 1 large organic head of broccoli, florets only
- Fresh Ginger
- 1 cup Coconut milk, boxed not canned
- 1 small onion diced
- 2 cloves of garlic minced
- 2 stalks celery diced
- 1 finger fresh turmeric
- 2 cups fresh kale, remove stems
- 3 cups of water
- ½ tsp. Himalayan salt and pepper to taste

1. In large pot add 3 cups of water, 1 small onion, 2 cloves of garlic, 2 stalks of celery and 1 finger of turmeric sliced. 4-6 fresh ginger slices. Add salt and pepper to taste. Bring to a boil. Add fresh kale. Add ½ the broccoli florets. Simmer until tender.
2. Remove the broth with the kale and florets and place in food processor to blend with 1 cup coconut milk. Blend well. Return it back to the pot. Add the remaining broccoli florets. Cook until tender.

Optional: Add cheese
       Sauerkraut
       Cayenne Pepper

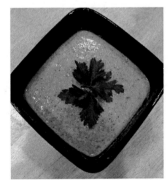

Apple Zucchini Rose

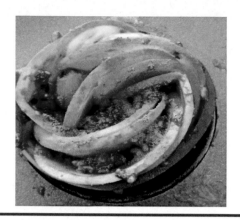

1. 2 organic zucchini, Slice long with a mandolin approx. ¼ inch thick. Lightly steam to soften. Do not overcook
2. 3 granny smith apples. Slice in crescent shape

   Filling: Combine in a food processor
3. 4 Medjool dates, pitted
4. ½ cup raspberries
5. ¼ tsp. nutmeg
6. ¼ tsp. cinnamon
7. 1 tsp. local honey

Lay the zucchini slices lengthwise on a cutting board and place your crescent apples about midway on the zucchini and line the apple across the length of it.
Add the date mixture in the middle where the zucchini and apples come together.

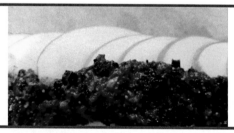

Gently roll the zucchini and apples strips to form a rose. Place them in a paper cupcake holder and then in a cupcake pan. Sprinkle cinnamon on top.
Bake at 350 for approx. 25 mins. Gently remove and enjoy!

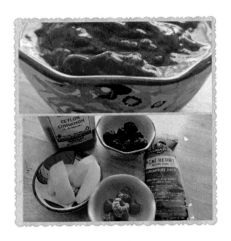

Acai and berry Sorbet

1. 1 pack frozen Acai
2. ½ organic apple
3. ½ cup of frozen black berries or blueberries
4. ¼ cup frozen raspberries
5. ½ teaspoon cinnamon
6. ¼ cup coconut milk or almond milk

Blend all ingredients in your vita mixer or food processor until smooth
Serve in ½ cup serving bowls.

Optional: Top with coconut, granola or chocolate chips

Notes:

_____

_____

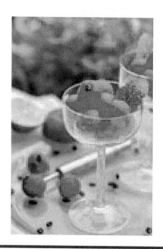

Watermelon Balls

Refreshing and yummy!

Scoop out watermelon in the shape of balls

Add:
Dash of Himalayan salt
Freshly chopped mint or basil
Fresh squeeze lime
Optional: A dash of oregano

A fully ripened watermelon is typically 6 percent sugar and 91 percent water by weight. Contains Vitamin C and very hydrating

NOTES: _____

_____

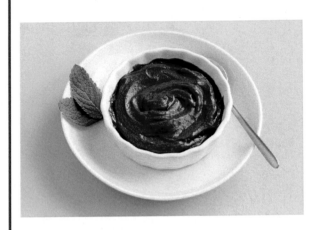

Raw Avocado Cacao Mousse

BEST MOUSSE – It's delicious! Guilt free too! Healthy fats from the avocado and coconut oil! Anti-oxidant from the raw cacao.

1. 1 Ripe Haas avocado
2. ¼ cup Raw Cacao (not cocoa)
3. 1 tsp. natural vanilla
4. 1 tsp. raw honey or maple syrup
5. 1 tbsp. raw coconut oil. (Hardened)
6. Optional ¼ cup blueberries, strawberries or raspberries blended with the avocado until smooth
7. Top with fresh fruit if desired or shavings of dark chocolate or nuts

Adjust the amount of raw cacao depending on your taste

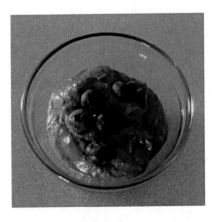

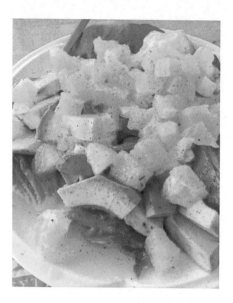

Avocado Mandarin Orange Salad

- 1-2 organic ripened Hass avocado
- 1-2 Mandarin Oranges or tangerines
- Romaine Lettuce
- 1 Fresh lemon
- Cayenne
- ½ teaspoon raw honey
- ½ teaspoon olive oil

1. Slice avocado in wedges
2. Dice oranges or tangerines
3. Lay avocado and oranges on a bed or romaine lettuce
4. Mix the juice of 1 freshly squeezed lemon with ½ teaspoon of raw honey and ½ teaspoon olive oil.
5. Drizzle dressing on the avocado mandarin salad
6. Sprinkle lightly with cayenne pepper
7. Chill and serve

NOTES: _____

_____

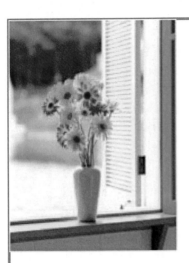

Journal Page

ABOUT GLORIA

Gloria Coppola has been in the healing arts for over 30 yrs. She is an intuitive holistic practitioner who has owned a massage school, wellness center and health food store. She attended Clayton School of Natural Healing, Hunter College and graduated from the Institute of Integrative Nutrition and Health Choices Healing Arts. Her passion for travel, healing and helping others has led her around the world to study with shaman, kahuna and many leading alternative teachers, including Deepak Chopra, David Wolfe, Dave Sandoval, Bernard Jensen, Caroline Myss to name a few.

Gloria is no stranger to the adversities of life, tragedy, stress and injury to her body. She understands pain, anxiety and depression. Her healing journey has taught her more compassion for others dealing with similar ailments. In 2005 she suffered a severe back injury at the same time menopause began. She was told she needed surgery or would not walk, however, she refused. The debilitating pain she suffered limited her once active and fit life. Weight became an issue for this once active happy lady. Tenacity, hope and faith led her to many healing arts practitioners, yogic practices, breathing techniques and finally to a super foods nutrition company. It was the right balance of nutrients that removed the inflammation, restored the strength in her spine, eliminated her depression and gave her a new life, one that would soon help thousands of others seeking help.

If you are reading this book today, you have stumbled upon a passionate woman who is on a mission to help others find a healthier lifestyle. Her dedication and commitment is unstoppable. Currently, 60 years young she is still learning and growing and has big dreams to be fulfilled.

Meet Gloria, she found a way and wants to share with anyone ready.

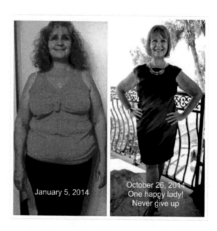

January 5, 2014

October 26, 2014
One happy lady!
Never give up

Alphabetical Index

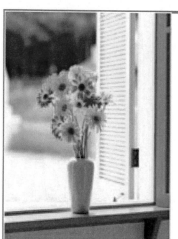

FINAL NOTES

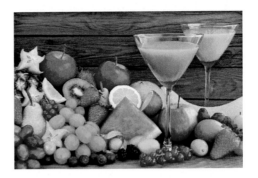

**Cheers to your
Lifestyle journey!**

I offer 3 and 6 months health-coaching programs for your continued success
www.GloriaCoppola.com

To learn more about detoxification programs or healthier nutritional supplementation along with meal planning please email me at
livegreenwithpurium@gmail.com

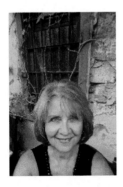

Exclusive Photography Credits 2016
Gloria Coppola
Licensed Stock Adobe
Licensed Microsoft Word

Gloria Coppola, Educator, author and
Certified Holistic Health & Lifestyle Coach

Made in the USA
San Bernardino, CA
18 April 2016